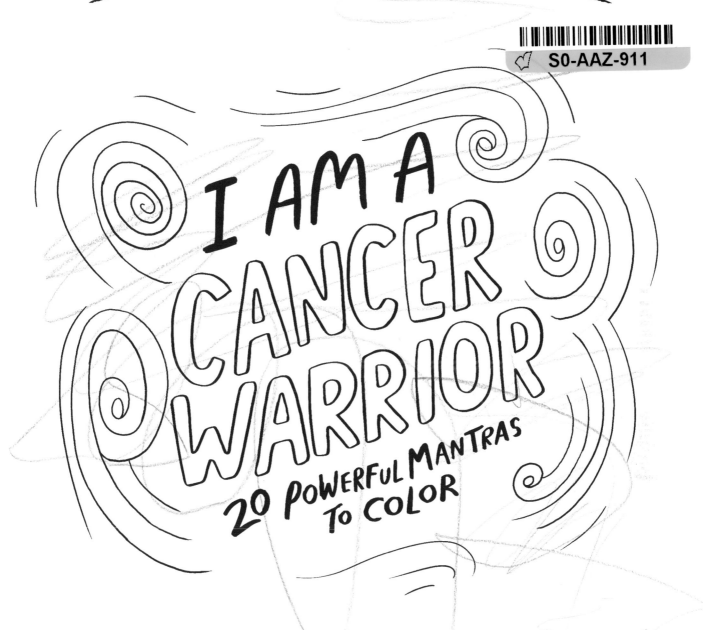

I Am A Cancer Warrior: 20 Powerful Mantras To Color © 2016 Kathy Weller.

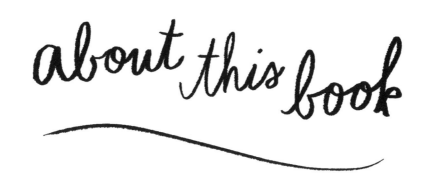

about this book

A member of my family got cancer a couple years ago. I really wanted to help in ways that were meaningful, practical, and tangible. But, I simply was not able to help out in many of the ways that I wanted to.

So, instead of lamenting on what I COULDN'T do, I thought about what I COULD do. I knew I could put my ART to good use to support him and lift his spirits!

Every day, for seven weeks of treatment, I sent a hand-drawn card in the mail. Each card had a different message of strength, support, solidarity, and often, humor! The phrases I wrote for those cards are very much like the ones in this book.

The cards were met with such gratitude and appreciation. I was overjoyed that I could help in a way that was really meaningful, personal, purposeful... and POWERFUL!

Eventually, I realized that I could also help others going through the same thing! And, the idea for this coloring book was born.

My hope is that this book will be a source of strength, empowerment, good energy and positive, healing vibes to YOU— strong Cancer Warriors, Survivors, family, and friends!!

KICK CANCER'S BUTT— UPSIDE DOWN, SIDEWAYS + INSIDE OUT!

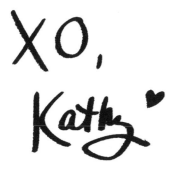

XO,
Kathy ♥

P.S. My relative is now thankfully cancer-free! YEAH!

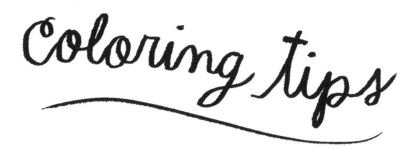

Coloring tips

 The paper in this book does well with dry media such as colored pencils, caran d'ache neocolor pastels, and other types of pastels and crayons.

 Markers of all types are fine to use, however, please place a page or two of plain paper underneath the page you are coloring to prevent bleed-through onto the next page.

 The coloring images are printed on one side of the paper, with the other side left intentionally blank.

 I made an effort to balance the design with a little extra space from the book binding. This was done to make it easier for you to cut the page out, if you wish to.

HAVE FUN + ENJOY YOURSELF!

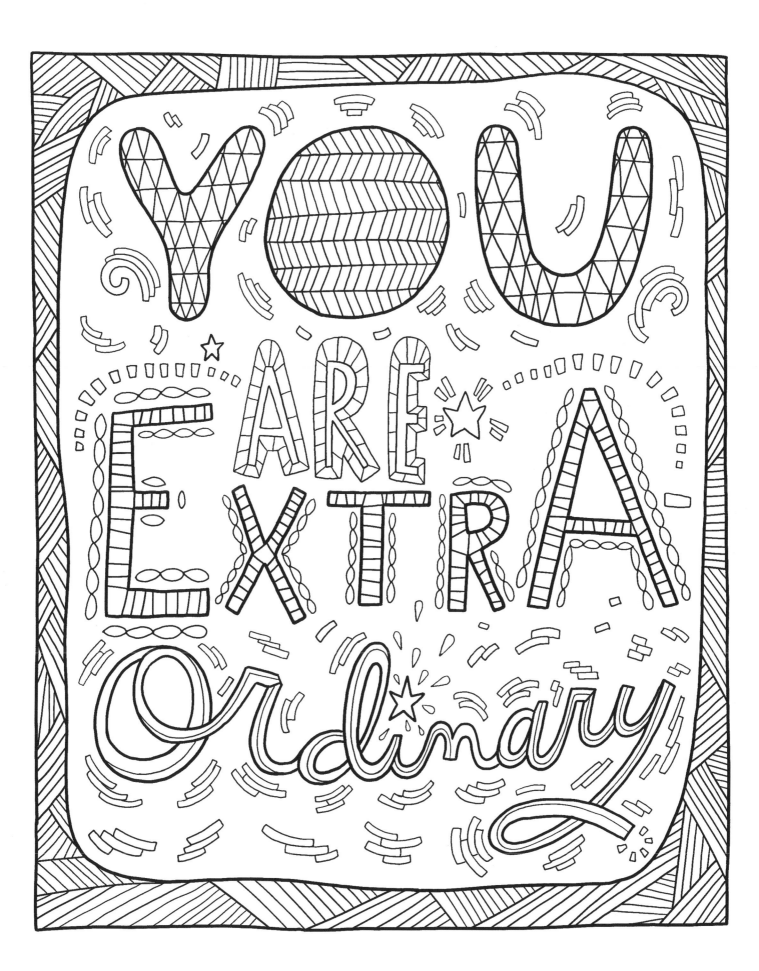

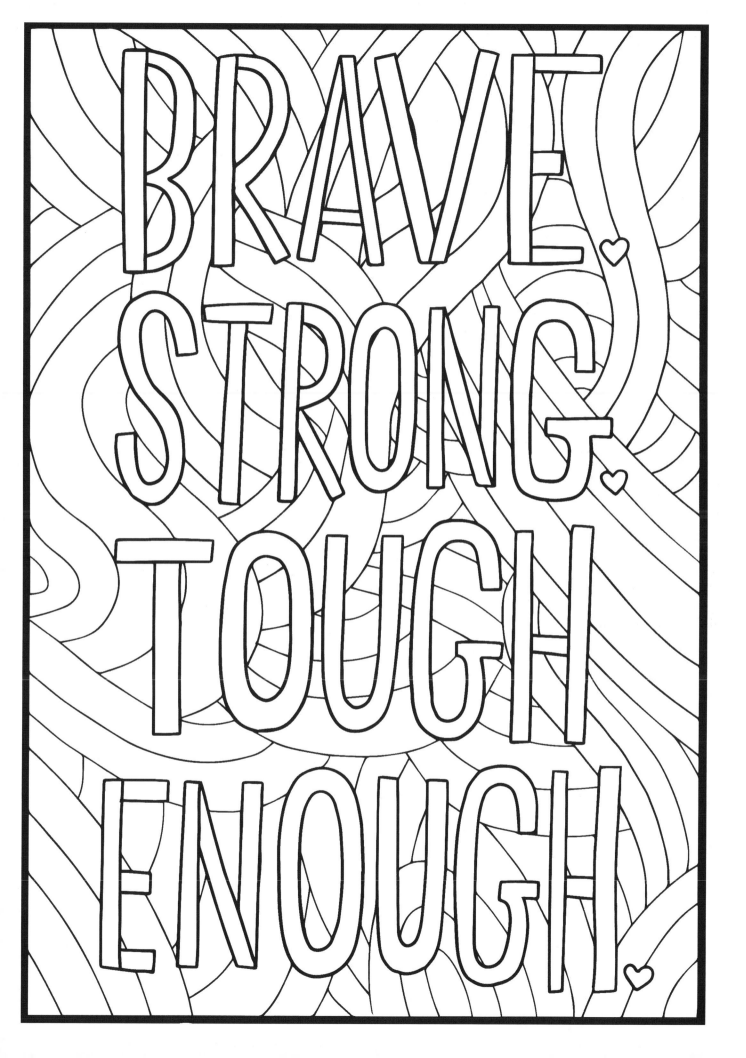

WHAT DOES NOT KILL US MAKES US STRONGER

nietzsche

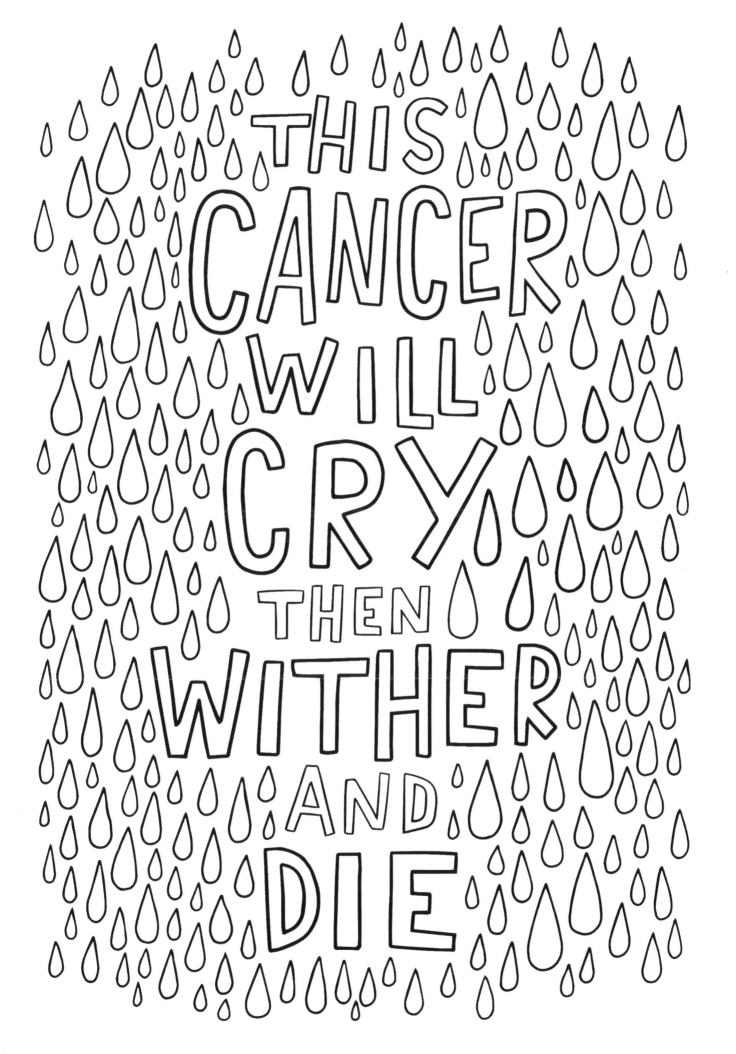

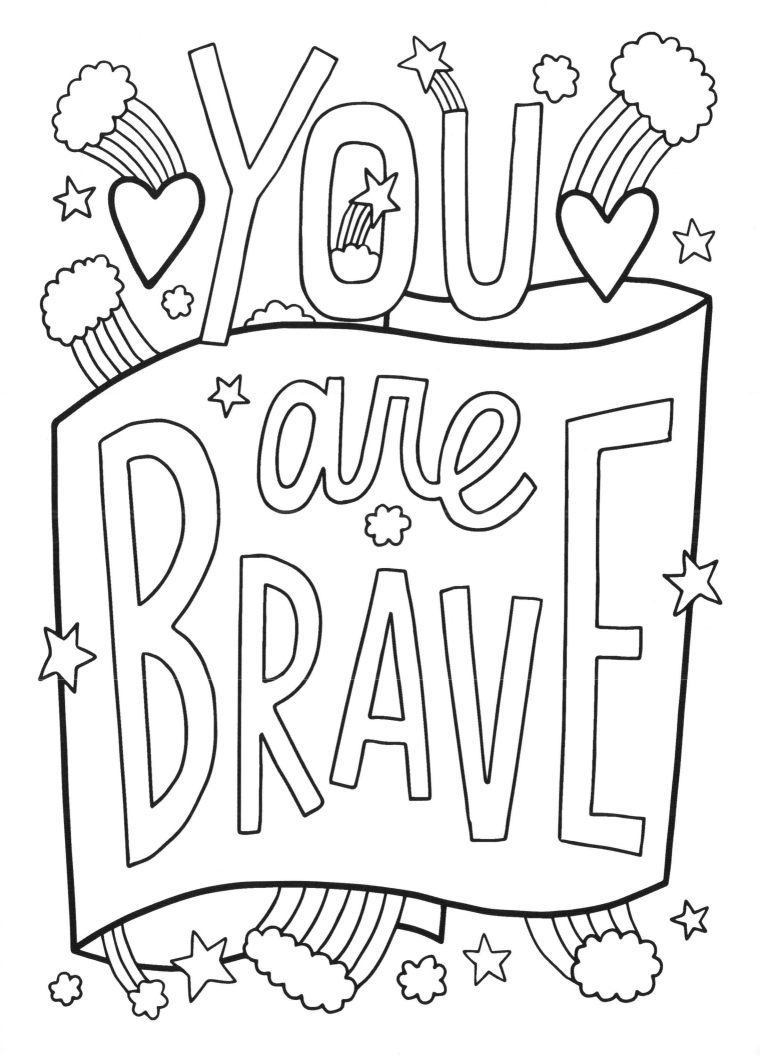

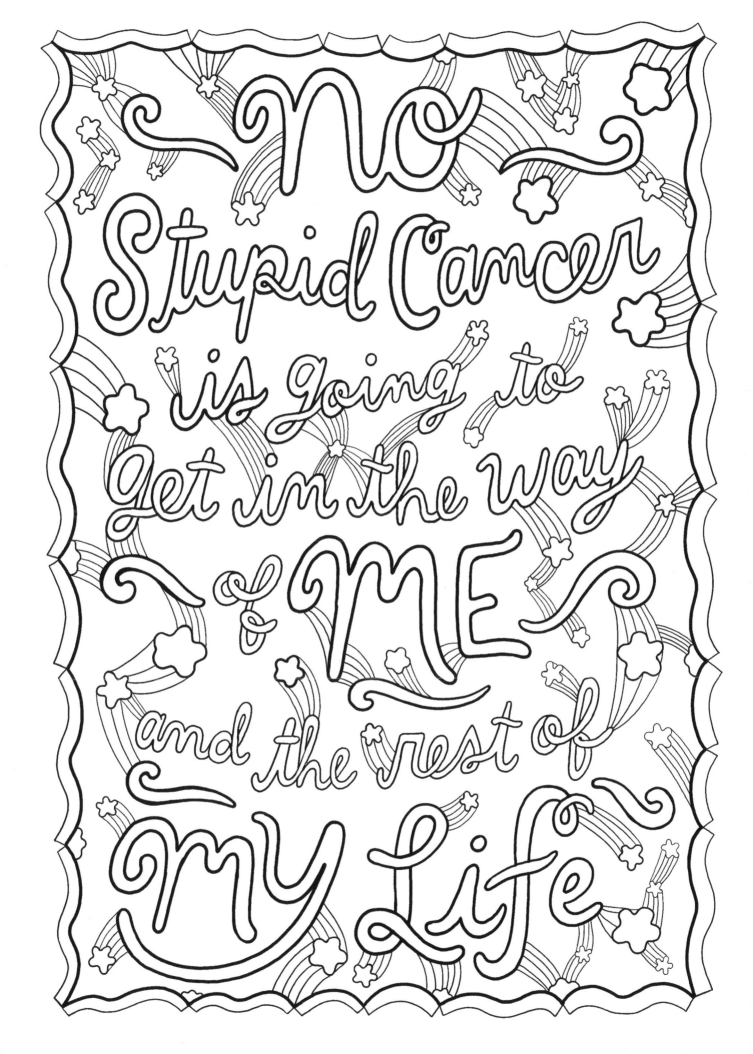

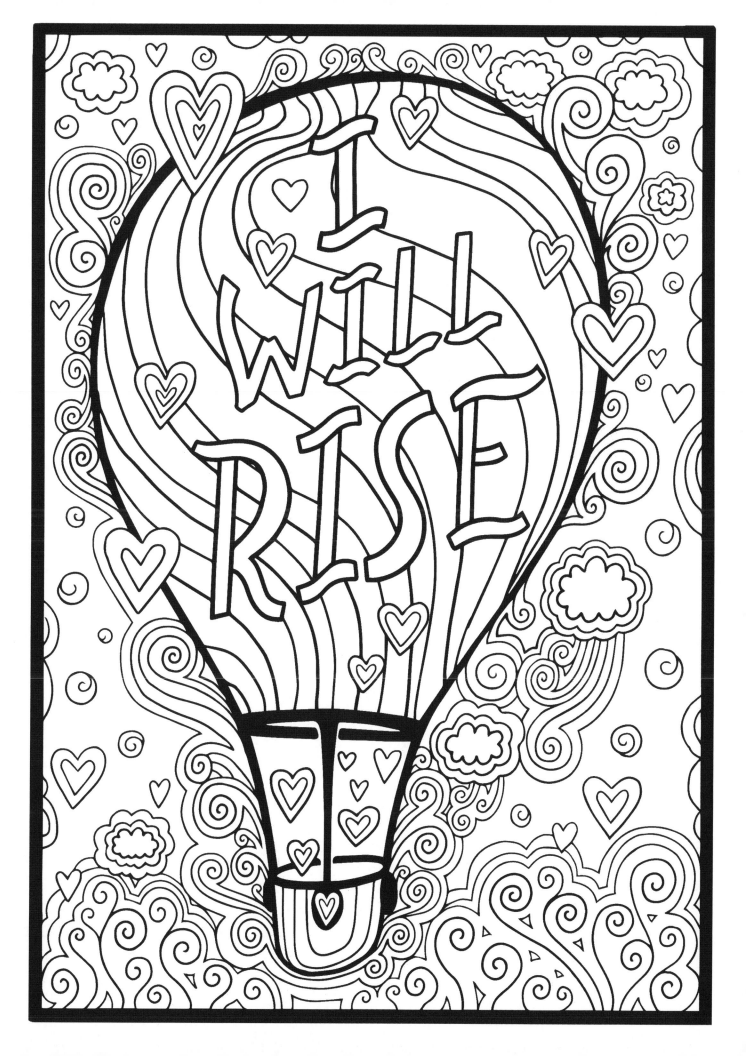

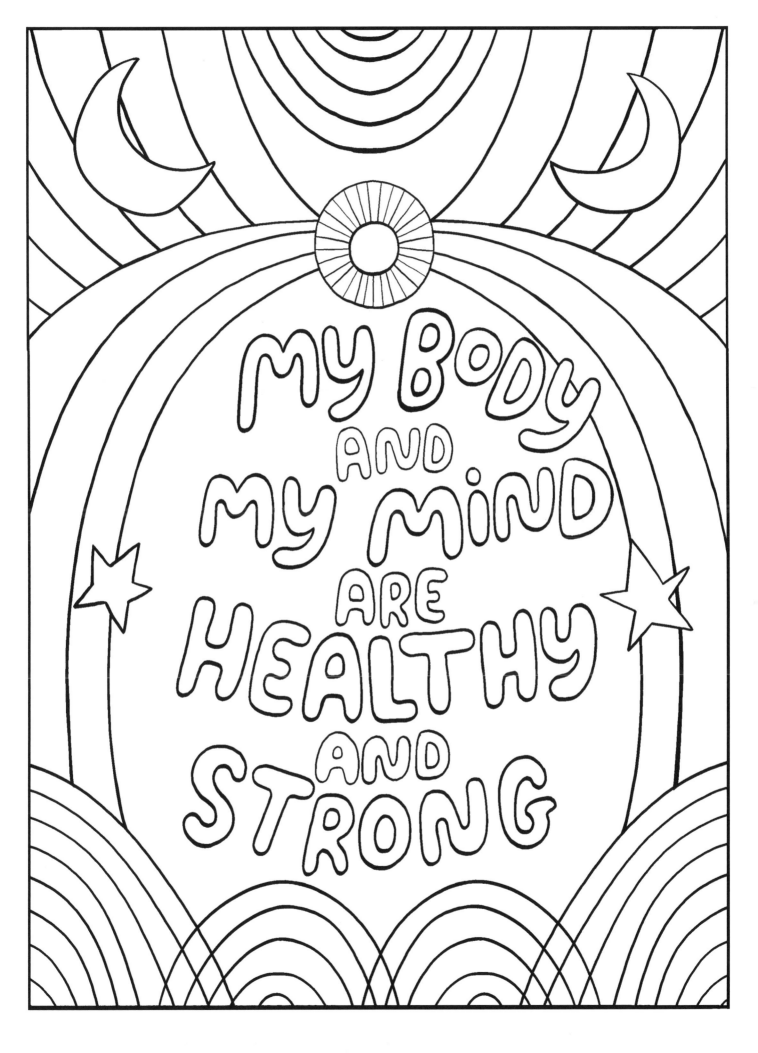

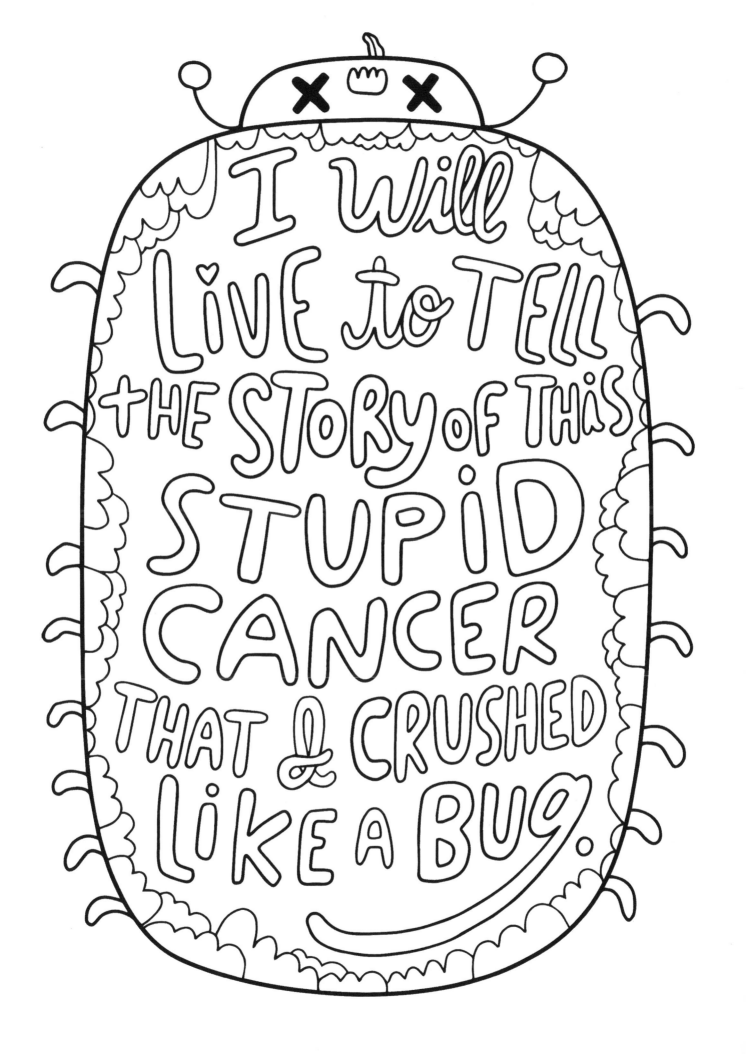

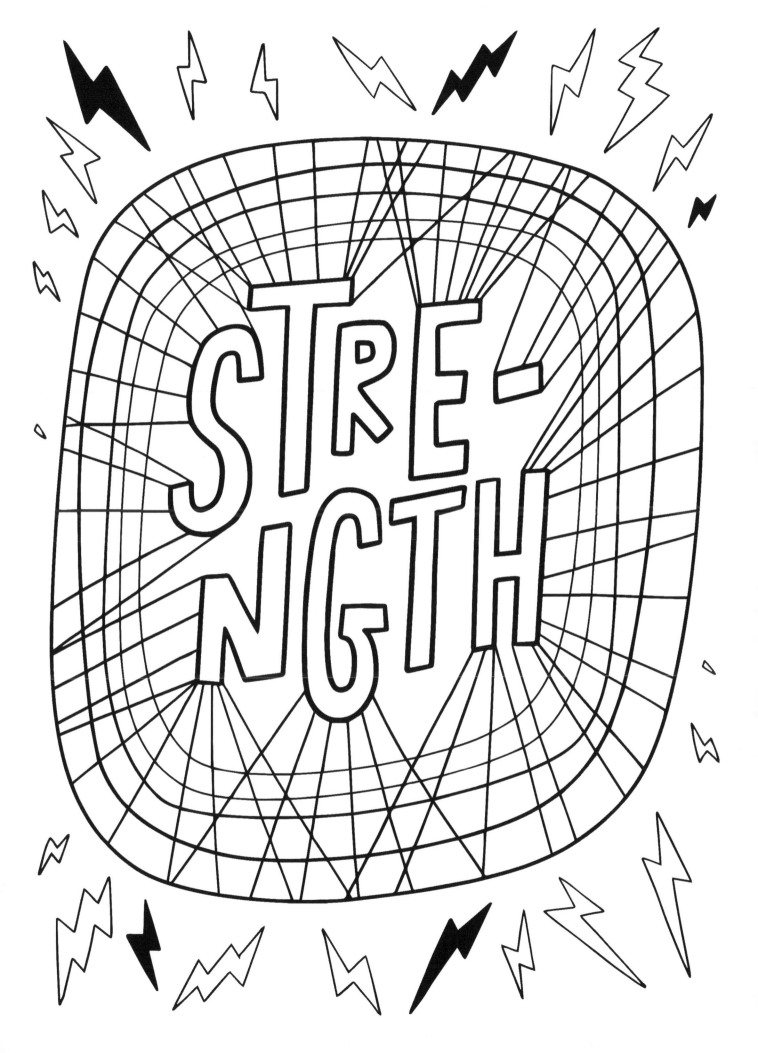

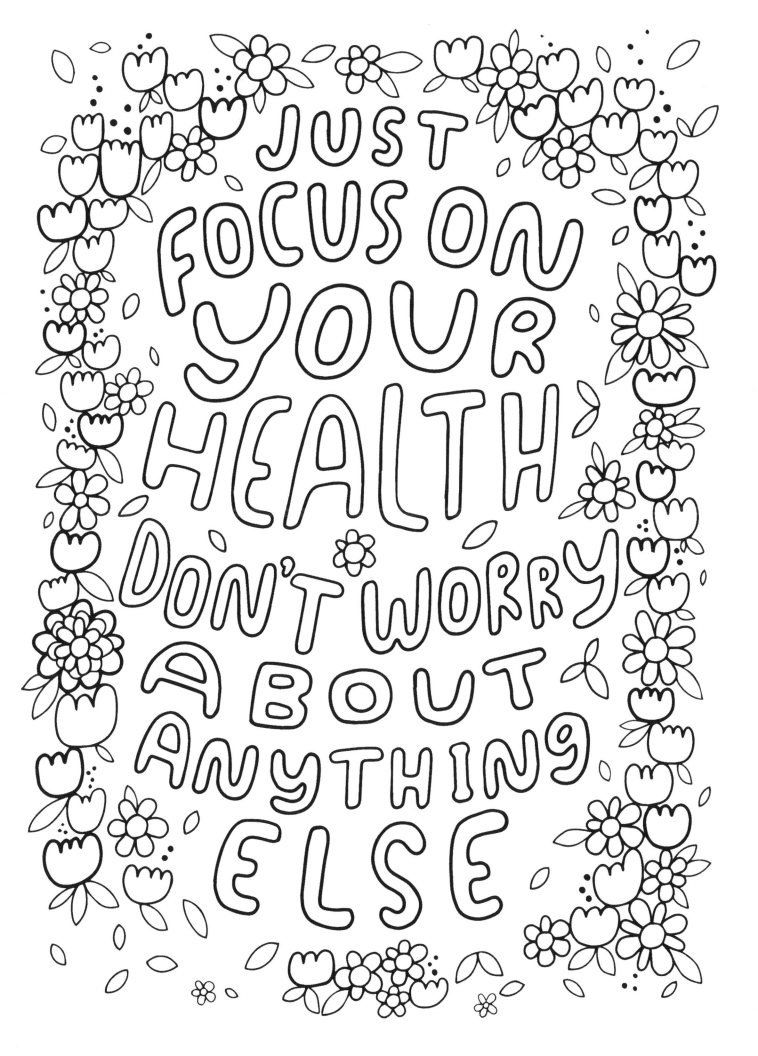

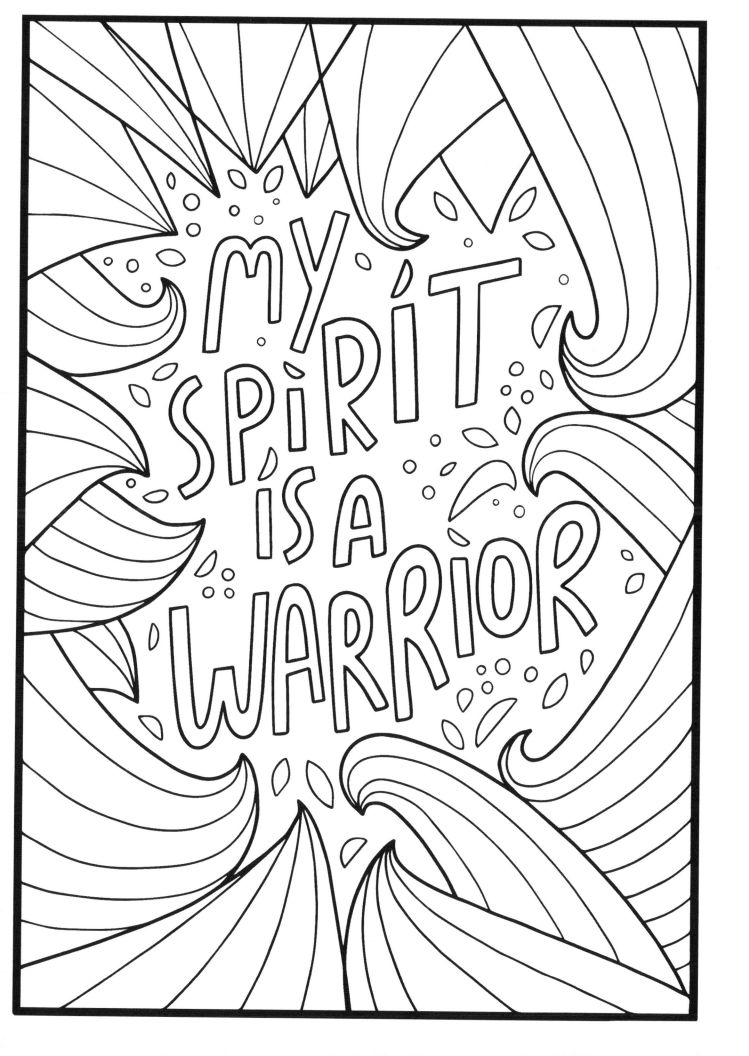

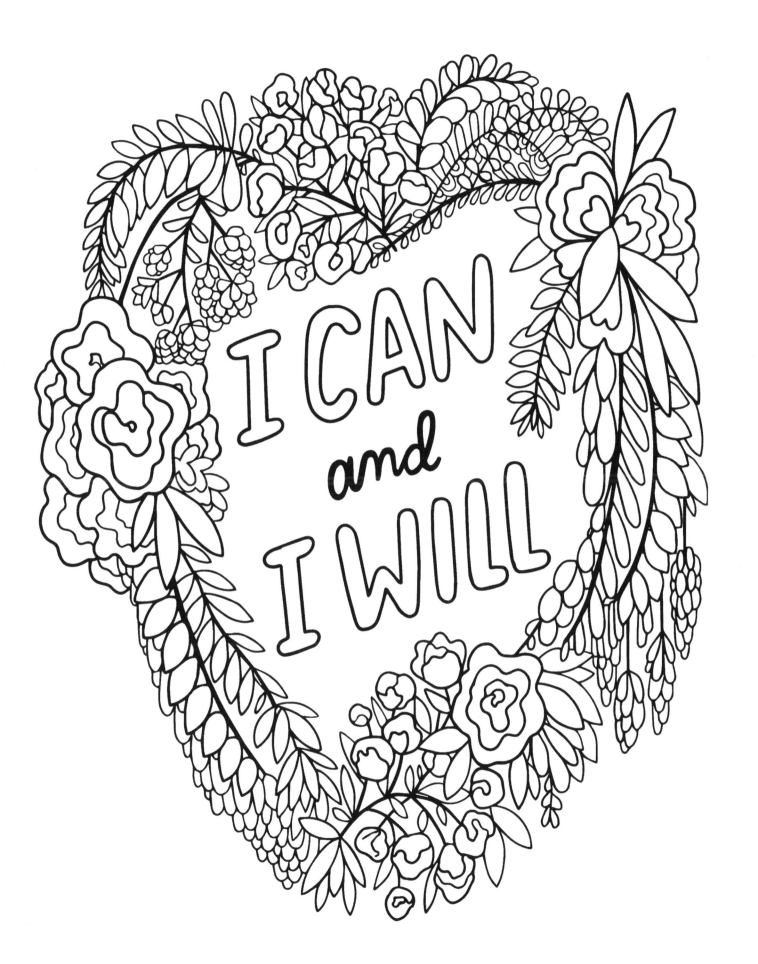

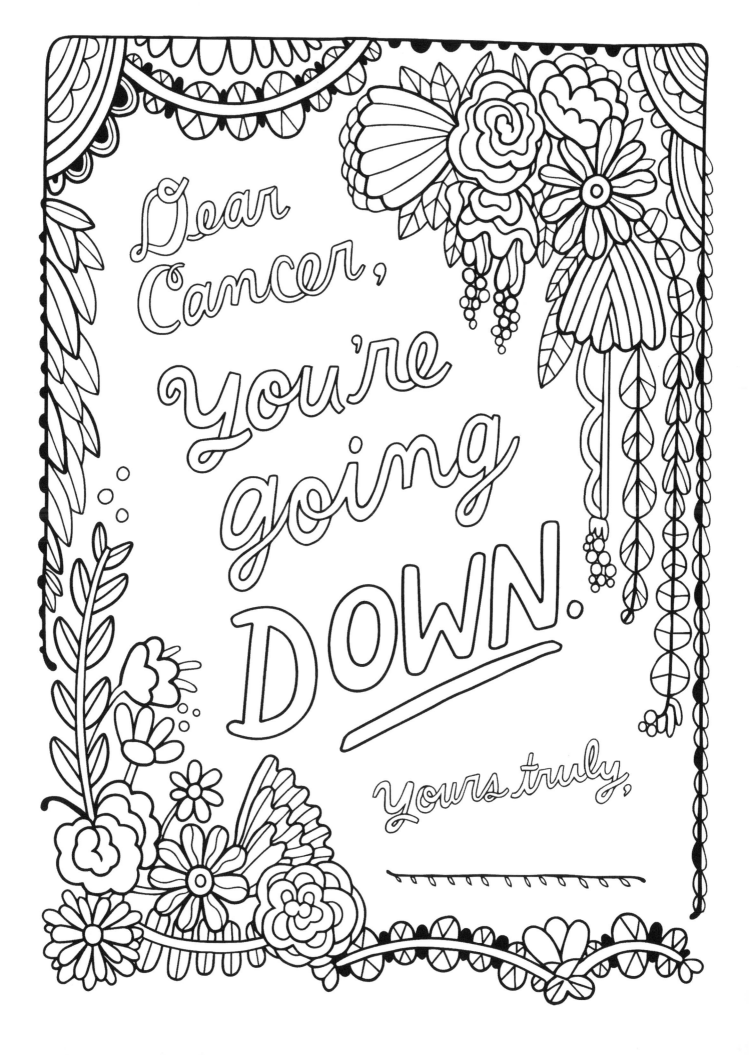

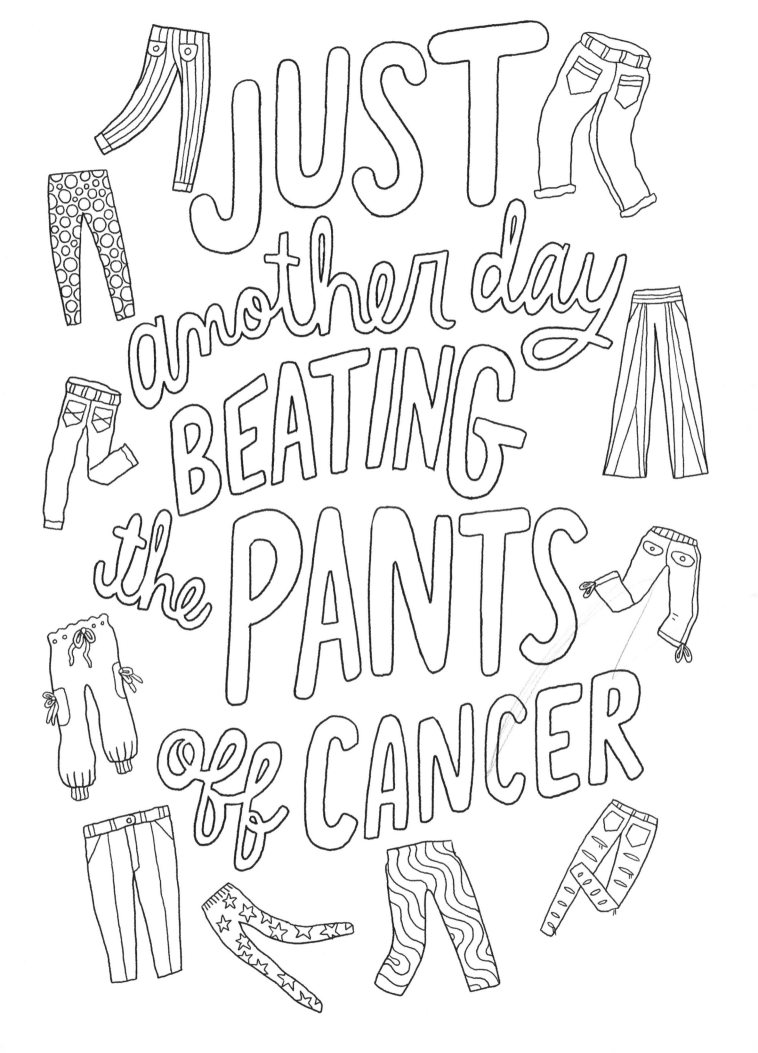

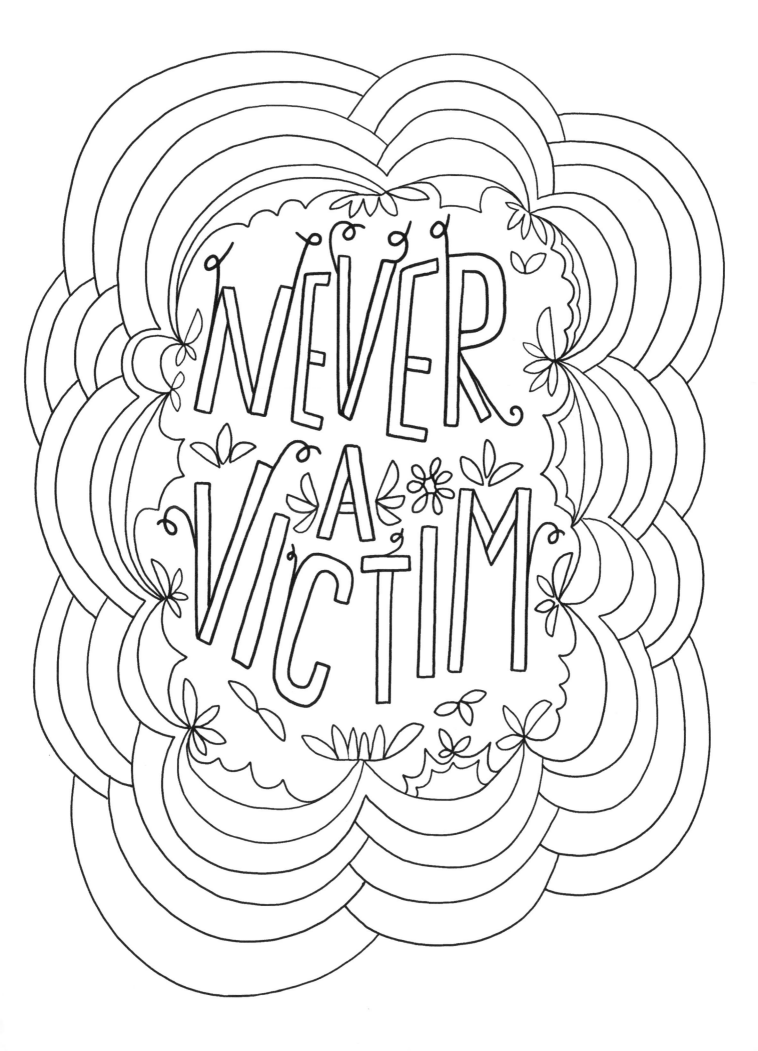

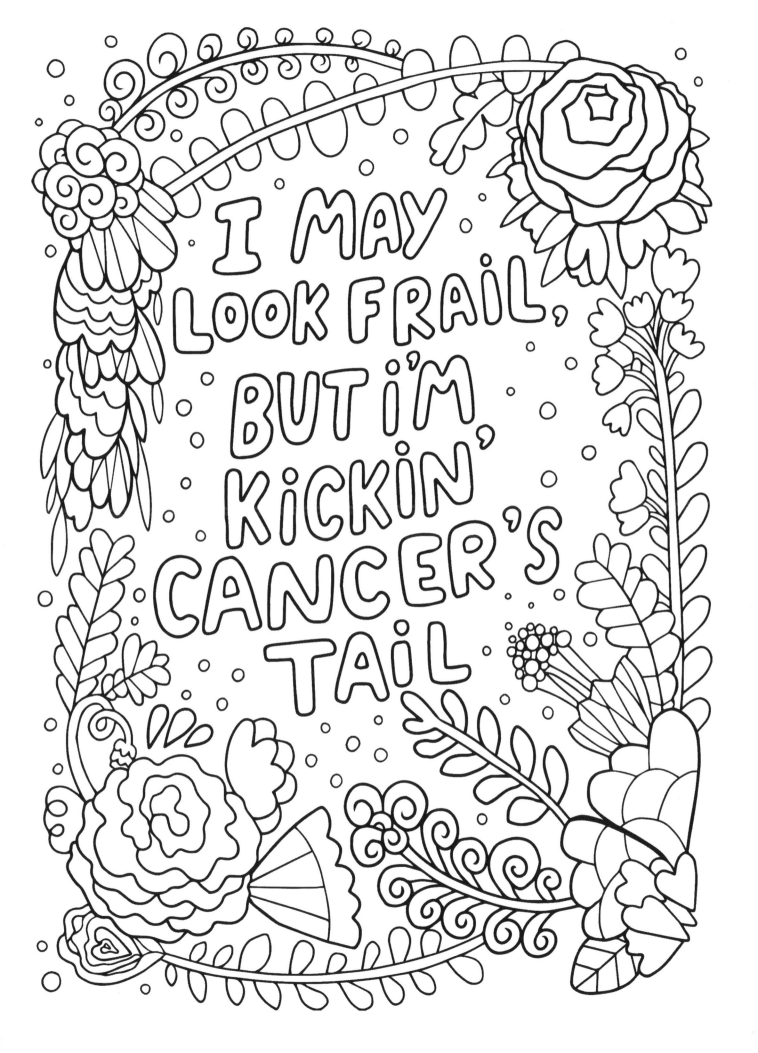

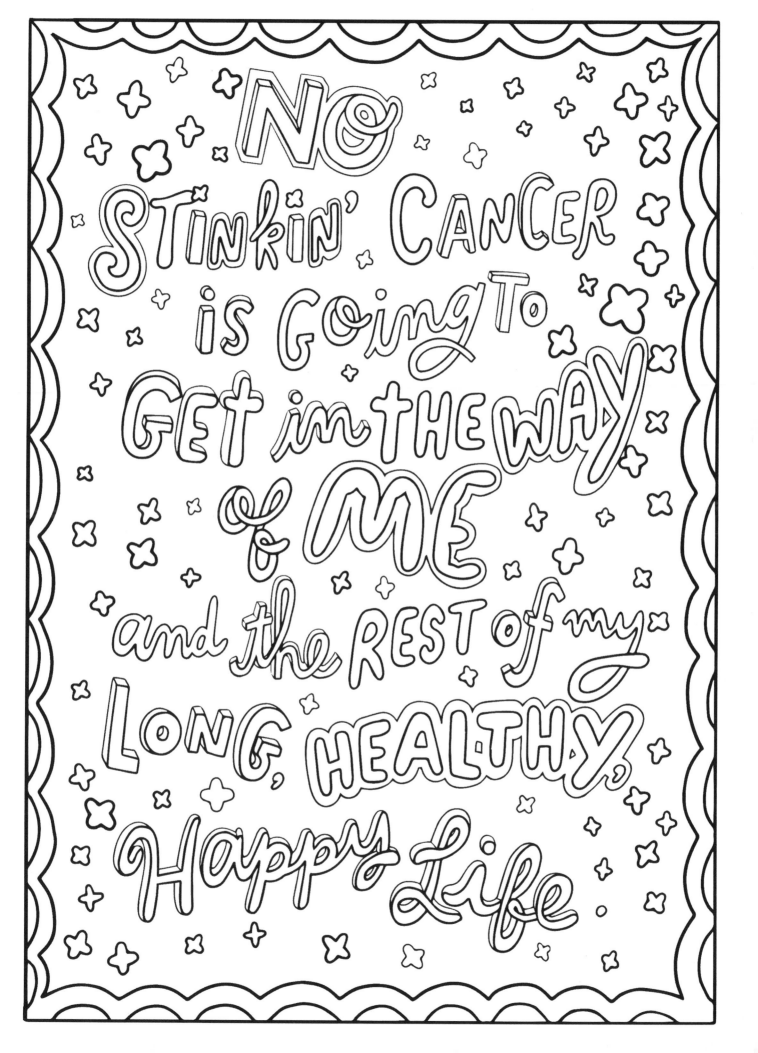

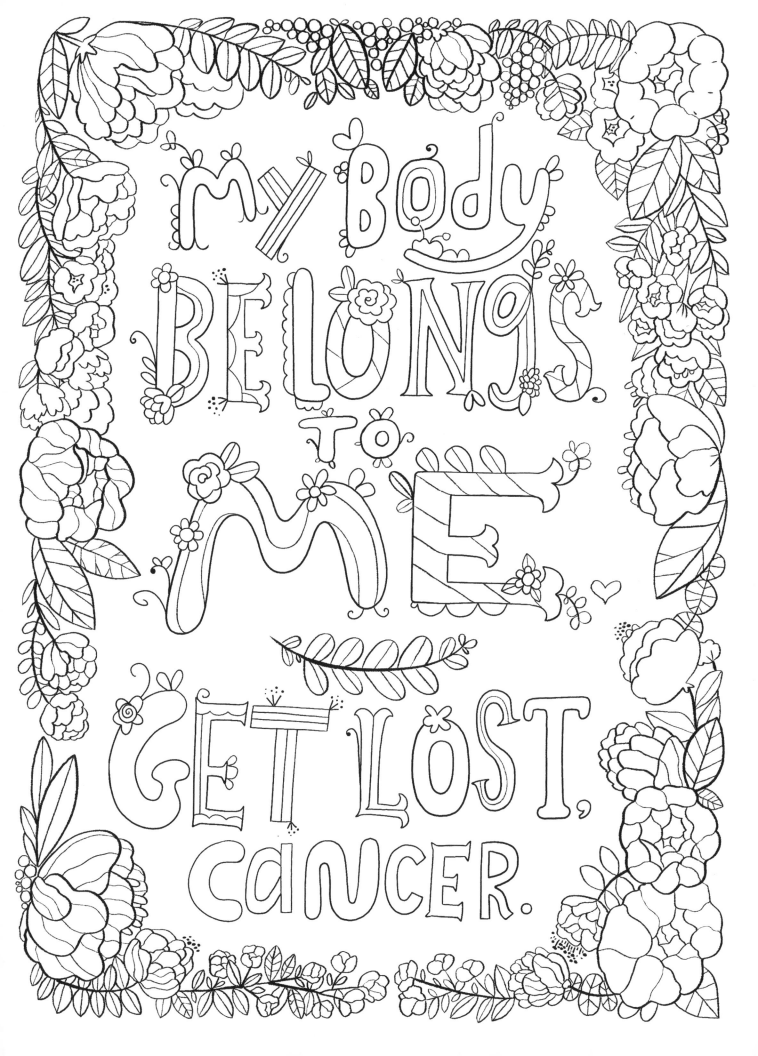

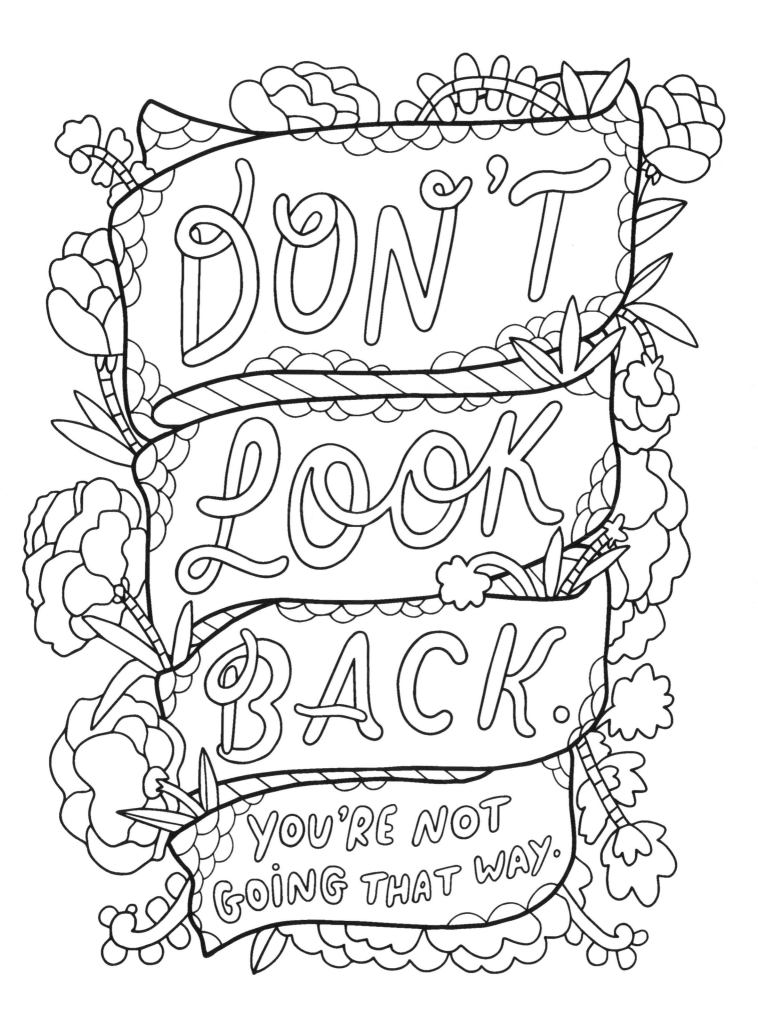

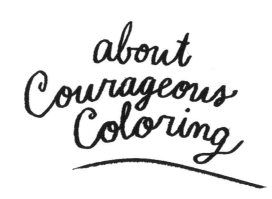

about Courageous Coloring

I started Courageous Coloring to encourage creative self-empowerment, exploration and discovery for everyone, without self-criticism or judgment. Experience creative motivation, inspiration, support and encouragement with Courageous Coloring!

If you are enjoying this book...

♥ **Please leave an Amazon review.**

♥ **People just like you are shopping Amazon right now, looking for a coloring book just like this!**

♥ **The more reviews this book has, the more visible Amazon will make it.**

♥ **Reviews with photos or videos of your beautiful coloring pages are extra, EXTRA-appreciated!!**

For latest releases, please visit:

CourageousColoring.com

let's connect!

Coloring books ♥ **courageouscoloring.com**

facebook ♥ facebook.com/**kathywellerart**

Twitter ♥ twitter.com/**kathywellerart**

Instagram ♥ instagram.com/**kathywellerart**

main site ♥ **kathyweller.com**

art videos ♥ youtube.com/**kathywellerart**

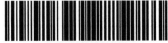

Made in the USA
Lexington, KY
26 March 2018